DEFEATING VISUAL IMPAIRMENT WITH EXPERT GUIDANCE

Ultimate Solution Handbook For Patients, Guardians Or Family To Understand, Manage, Treat, Prevent, Reverse Symptoms And Live Well

DR. POTTER WHITLEY

DISCLAIMER

This book's contents are meant to be used solely for informative purposes. The information should not be used as a replacement for expert medical advice, diagnosis, or care.

The information contained in this book is accurate and reliable, having been verified by the author to the best of his ability. Nevertheless, the author disclaims all express and implied representations and warranties regarding the availability, correctness, appropriateness, completeness, and reliability of the material provided here. You bear full responsibility for any reliance you may have on such material.

For informational purposes, this book may make reference to or mention of certain people, things, websites, organizations, or other names. The author has no connection to, endorsement from, or recommendation for these organizations. The author's approval or validation is not implied by the inclusion of these references.

Any direct, indirect, incidental, special, or consequential damages resulting from using or not being able to use the material in this book are not covered by the author's liability policy. For medical advice and counsel particular to their circumstances, readers are advised to check with experienced healthcare specialists.

The content, materials, and information in this book are subject to change at any time without prior notice, at the author's discretion. The text may contain errors or omissions for which the author is not responsible.

By reading this book, you understand and accept the conditions of this disclaimer.

THE REASON BEHIND THIS BOOK

Regarding vision impairment, "Defeating VISUAL IMPAIRMENT With Expert Guidance" is an invaluable source of information and assistance. The numerous dimensions of this difficult illness are illuminated as this book explores its complex facets. This book's goal—illuminating the value of professional assistance in negotiating the intricacies of visual impairment—is highlighted in the Introduction, which also sets the scene by examining the backdrop.

Sections that follow provide a thorough and informative examination of vision impairment. In addition to exploring the causes and risk factors, it clarifies the terminology and types of visual impairment and persuasively describes the significant impact it has on day-to-day life. Experts in the field are acknowledged in this book, with ophthalmologists, optometrists, rehabilitation specialists, assistive technology specialists, educators, and support personnel all receiving special recognition for their valuable contributions.

An important part of the process is Diagnosis and Assessment, which elaborates on the diagnostic methods and instruments used while highlighting the significance of early detection. As a complete resource for those suffering from visual impairment, the treatment options included in the following chapters include medicinal interventions, surgical procedures, vision rehabilitation programs, and therapeutic techniques.

In addition to providing diagnosis and therapy, "Defeating Visual Impairment With Expert Guidance" delves deeply into assistive technology. With hope and useful answers, this book presents a realistic picture of the modern scene, including screen readers, Braille displays, applications, smart gadgets, and magnification software.

Acknowledging the significance of classroom accommodations, adaptive learning materials, specialist teaching strategies, and inclusive education, educational support and inclusive practices receive the attention they merit.

Sensitively examining the psychological effects of vision impairment, coping mechanisms are provided to create a strong support network.

In addition to theory, this book offers practical advice on how people with visual impairments can live freely. People are given comprehensive support to lead happy lives through the provision of adaptive living skills, orientation and mobility training, house modifications, and career and employment coaching.

This book motivates me by showcasing positive experiences and inspirational adventures. The platform provides biographical information about individuals who have overcome visual impairment and highlights their accomplishments in diverse fields. Progress in medical research, new assistive technologies, and potential teaching methods are all anticipated by the investigation of future trends and research.

"Visual impairment defeated with professional advice" is a monument to tenacity, intelligence, and advancement.

It provides more than simply facts for individuals coping with visual impairment; its captivating story and affirmation of the human spirit make it an invaluable resource that can help them achieve success.

TABLE OF CONTENT

TABLE OF CONTENT

CHAPTER ONE

OVERVIEW
History:

For millions of people worldwide, visual impairment is a major obstacle that affects their everyday lives and prevents them from taking advantage of many opportunities. From partial sight to total blindness, this ailment includes a range of visual impairments. Congenital disorders, degenerative diseases, trauma, and aging-related factors are some of the reasons for vision impairment. A ray of hope has recently emerged for those with vision impairments because of technical developments and therapeutic therapies. It may be somewhat daunting for individuals and their families to sort through the plethora of information and approaches that are accessible.

"Defeating VISUAL IMPAIRMENT With Expert Guidance" was inspired by the urgent need for a thorough and approachable manual to assist those who are struggling with vision loss. By providing a comprehensive approach that covers the emotional and psychological components of vision impairment in addition to its physical features, this book seeks to be a beacon of knowledge and support. A fuller awareness of the difficulties experienced by people with visual impairments and the changing field of technologies and therapies aimed at improving their quality of life can be attained by readers by exploring the history of visual impairment.

The Goal Of This Book

"Defeating VISUAL IMPAIRMENT With Expert Guidance" aims to strengthen the quality of life of people who are visually impaired by providing them and their support systems with the information and resources they need. As a complete resource, the book aims to provide insights into all facets of living with vision impairment, from short-term difficulties to long-term plans for success in both personal and professional spheres. To help people with visual impairments feel less alone and more confident about their options for support, it aims to close the information gap.

The book strives to instill resilience and confidence in its readers by combining personal narratives, professional insights, and helpful advice. With a roadmap that points the way to a more fulfilling life, it aims to be a guide for individuals navigating the challenges of visual impairment. The book establishes a path that seeks empowerment, self-discovery, and a sense of community rather than just survival by plainly stating the goal.

Why Professional Advice Is Important

The process of overcoming vision impairment is greatly aided by expert guidance. Professional experience in the industry is becoming more and more valuable as technology keeps developing and therapeutic approaches get more complex. ophthalmologists, rehabilitation specialists, assistive technology specialists, and psychologists are among the professionals who specialize in different aspects of visual impairment and whose advice is highly recommended in this book.

Under the direction of an expert, people can be certain to receive individualized and focused support in addition to precise information about their illness. Experts in the sector can provide individuals and their families with emotional support, suggestions for the newest assistive devices, and customized daily life tactics. Within the framework of a holistic approach to well-being, the book delves into the need to collaborate with specialists to build a connection that extends beyond prescription medicine.

In summary, "Defeating VISUAL IMPAIRMENT With Expert Guidance" seeks to empower and educate those who are affected by visual impairment, serving as a light of hope. An extensive examination of the many facets of living with vision impairment is made possible by the introduction, which explores the history of visual impairment, states the goal of the book, and emphasizes the value of professional advice.

CHAPTER TWO

BEING AWARE OF VISUAL IMPAIRMENT
Visual Impairment Definition and Types:

Any degree of vision loss that adversely affects a person's capacity to perceive and comprehend visual information is collectively referred to as visual impairment. Knowing that vision impairment can take many different forms and does not always result in total blindness is important. A person with low vision, reduced visual acuity absolute blindness, or no awareness of light, are at opposite ends of the spectrum.

Tasks requiring specific visual information are difficult to do when one has low vision, which is commonly defined as a considerable decline in visual acuity. Ocular degeneration, diabetic retinopathy, and glaucoma are a few disorders that may cause this. Total blindness, which can be caused by catastrophic accidents, degenerative diseases, or congenital abnormalities, is on the other extreme of the spectrum and denotes the absence of visual perception.

Loss of peripheral vision is another way that visual impairment can appear, making it challenging to move around without getting lost. A condition that narrows the field of vision is retinitis pigmentosa. Making assistance and interventions more individualized to fit the unique requirements of people with various visual problems requires an understanding of the many types of visual impairment.

Risk Factors And Causes:

A multitude of reasons, including acquired illnesses, age-related changes, and congenital factors, can lead to visual impairment. Genetic problems, prenatal virus exposure, or anomalies in the development of the visual system are examples of congenital causes. Infections, trauma, or illnesses such as diabetic retinopathy, glaucoma, or cataracts are examples of acquired causes.

In elderly populations, problems like cataracts and macular degeneration are more common, which means that age-related variables have a major role in visual impairment. Lens deterioration can also be caused by environmental causes, like extended exposure to UV radiation or work-related risks. Lifestyle decisions such as smoking and eating poorly can raise the chance of illnesses developing that cause vision impairment.

Preventive actions and early intervention depend on an understanding of the causes and risk factors. There is a considerable reduction in the chance of visual impairment with regular eye exams, healthy living, and eye injury prevention methods.

Influence on Day-to-Day Living:

The deterioration of one's vision has a significant impact on many facets of an individual's life, including social interactions, education, mobility, and independence. It becomes harder for people with visual impairments to navigate the physical world because they can have trouble identifying landmarks and overcoming obstacles. Adaptive techniques and assistive technology are needed when simple tasks like writing, reading, and object identification become difficult.

Because people may need help from others to complete everyday tasks, independence is frequently impaired. Without the right assistance and accommodations, employment prospects would be scarce, and academic goals might be hampered. Facial expressions and nonverbal clues—which are crucial for effective communication—may become harder to read in social situations.

Offering complete support systems is one way to address how visual impairment affects day-to-day living. Assistive technology integration, accommodations for learning, and physical accessibility features are all included in this. Notwithstanding the difficulties presented by vision impairment, rehabilitation programs, and adaptive skills training are essential in enabling people to navigate and engage fully in daily life.

CHAPTER THREE

VISUAL IMPAIRMENT EXPERTS' ROLE
Professionals In Ophthalmology And Optometry:

Due to their specialization in the diagnosis and treatment of eye disorders, optometrists and ophthalmologists are essential in the fight against visual impairment. Primary vision care is the domain of optometrists, who are medical professionals with training in primary care, and ophthalmologists, who specialize in eye care. For the early diagnosis and treatment of vision problems, these professionals are indispensable. They can detect several types of eye conditions, including glaucoma, cataracts, and retinal illnesses, by doing thorough eye exams.

Ophthalmologists handle conditions that, if left untreated, could result in blindness to fight visual impairment. Significant improvements in vision restoration are possible with procedures including cataract surgery, corneal transplants, and retinal operations. When it comes to helping people with visual impairments make the most of their residual vision, optometrists provide low-vision aids and corrective lenses.

Moreover, a multidisciplinary strategy for managing vision impairment is created by these professionals working in conjunction with other specialists. Patients who are at risk of visual impairment or who are already having vision problems should see ophthalmologists and optometrists regularly. This is because prompt treatment can stop more damage from occurring and improve general eye health.

Experts in Rehabilitation:

The ability of people with visual impairments to live autonomous and meaningful lives is greatly enhanced by rehabilitation specialists. These professionals teach people how to comfortably navigate their surroundings. They are frequently trained in mobility and orientation.

To properly use alternative senses, such as a white cane or guide dog for mobility, they offer persons useful skills.

Rehab specialists also concentrate on improving activities of daily living. ADLs (activities of daily living) such as cleaning, cooking, and personal hygiene are among the things that can be taught to people with visual impairments. The general well-being and independence of people with visual impairments are greatly enhanced by rehabilitation specialists' provision of useful skills.

In addition, these professionals deal with the emotional and psych

ological effects of vision loss. Rehabilitative professionals provide counseling and support to help people negotiate the emotional obstacles of coping with eyesight loss. Rehabilitators enable people to overcome obstacles and lead fulfilling lives despite visual impairments by using a holistic approach.

Professionals in Assistive Technology:

Through the utilization of technology, assistive technology specialists significantly contribute to the defeat of vision impairment. These experts are focused on locating and putting into practice digital solutions that meet the unique requirements of people who are blind or visually impaired. With the use of assistive technology, people with visual impairments can access a vast array of options, including braille displays, screen readers, software for magnification, and speech-to-text.

The function that assistive technology plays in employment and education is one of its major contributions. This field's experts collaborate closely with businesses and schools to include technology that improves job performance and learning. Specialized software and gadgets can provide equal educational opportunities for visually impaired pupils by leveling the playing field. Likewise, assistive technology makes it possible for people to succeed in their chosen fields of work by offering resources that meet their vision requirements.

In addition, professionals in assistive technology are always conducting research and development to stay up to date on the most recent developments. This guarantees the availability of state-of-the-art solutions for people with visual impairments, thereby enhancing their quality of life. When it comes to making the world more inclusive and accessible for people with visual impairments, assistive technology specialists play an increasingly important role as technology advances.

Support Personnel and Teachers:

Teachers and support personnel play a vital role in the academic and social development of people with visual impairments when it comes to the fight against visual impairment. These specialists are vital to the establishment of learning and development environments since they frequently operate in inclusive classes or specialized institutions.

To accommodate different learning styles, teachers modify their teaching strategies, resulting in a customized education for children with visual impairments. Education can be made more accessible by utilizing a variety of resources, including audio resources, tactile learning materials, and braille instruction. To develop an all-encompassing and encouraging learning environment, educators also work in conjunction with other experts, such as mobility and orientation teachers and assistive technology specialists.

Additional support is given to students with visual impairments by support professionals, such as resource experts and teaching assistants. To help students feel like they belong in the school community, they coordinate inclusive activities, provide one-on-one support, and assist with navigation. This teamwork-based method fosters social integration, emotional health, and academic performance simultaneously.

Advocating for the needs of students with visual impairments is a critical duty that educators and support workers undertake. Through fostering inclusivity and increasing awareness, they help to build a diverse educational environment where all students, regardless of visual ability, can succeed.

Ultimately, the collaborative endeavors of ophthalmologists, optometrists, rehabilitation specialists, assistive technology specialists, educators, and support personnel culminate in a complete and synergistic strategy to tackle visual impairment. With a shared objective of enabling people with visual impairments to live happy, independent lives, professional groups each contribute special talents and competence to the table. These professionals have a significant impact on changing the lives of people with visual impairments by providing early intervention, adaptive technologies, rehabilitation services, and inclusive education.

CHAPTER FOUR

DIAGNOSIS AND ASSESSMENT
Importance of Early Detection:

For prompt management to be possible and any problems to be avoided, early recognition of visual impairment is essential. Undiagnosed visual impairment can have a major negative effect on a person's quality of life by making it more difficult for them to learn, interact with others, and carry out daily tasks. Early detection is especially important in youngsters as eyesight is so important to their whole development. Undiagnosed visual problems can cause social and scholastic problems.

Furthermore, early detection makes it possible to identify disorders that may be treated and may be the cause of visual impairment. With prompt intervention, certain eye disorders, such as refractive defects or specific eye illnesses, can be effectively controlled or repaired. Healthcare practitioners can prescribe glasses, offer vision therapy, or suggest other suitable steps to address the underlying causes of visual impairment by spotting these problems early on.

When it comes to stopping the advancement of eye conditions like glaucoma, macular degeneration, or diabetic retinopathy in adults, early detection becomes essential. Routine eye exams are essential for early detection of these disorders since they frequently develop slowly and without symptoms in their early stages. Vision preservation and halting more degeneration can be achieved by quickly identifying and treating these disorders.

Furthermore, early identification improves public health by lessening the financial burden of untreated vision impairment. Early detection and treatment can lower the cost of treating advanced eye disorders as well as the negative social effects of vision impairment, such as decreased productivity and increased dependency.

In conclusion, early detection is critical to the fight against visual impairment since it can save long-term difficulties, improve overall quality of life, and lessen the financial and social costs of untreated vision issues.

Instruments and Methods for Diagnosis:

To effectively assess the health and performance of the visual system, a variety of sophisticated diagnostic tools and techniques are needed for an effective diagnosis of visual impairment. To assess various facets of vision and eye health, optometrists and ophthalmologists use a range of tools and techniques.

The visual acuity test, which gauges visual clarity at different distances, is one of the basic diagnostic instruments. This examination, which is frequently done with the aid of an eye chart, can identify refractive defects such as astigmatism, hyperopia, and myopia. The slit-lamp biomicroscope, which enables eye care specialists to assess the anterior section of the eye, including the cornea, iris, and lens, is another crucial diagnostic tool.

Optical coherence tomography (OCT) has emerged as a vital diagnostic tool for a thorough evaluation of the retina. OCT helps with the detection and treatment of several retinal disorders, including diabetic retinopathy and macular degeneration, by providing high-resolution cross-sectional photographs of the retinal layers.

Perimetry is used in situations when visual field flaws need to be assessed. The purpose of this test is to map out the patient's visual field and identify any irregularities that may indicate glaucoma or other diseases. Tonometry also monitors intraocular pressure, which is important in the diagnosis and follow-up of glaucoma.

Advances in imaging technologies, including fundus photography and fluorescein angiography, have improved eye care practitioners' diagnostic abilities in recent years. With the use of these instruments, a variety of retinal illnesses can be diagnosed by providing thorough recording and examination of the fundus and retinal vasculature.

In addition to facilitating accurate diagnosis, the use of modern diagnostic technologies allows medical personnel to customize treatment programs to meet the specific needs of each patient. Frequent upgrades and the use of new technologies enhance the diagnostic methods for overcoming visual impairment.

Entire Visual Evaluation:

A thorough assessment of the visual system's components, such as visual acuity, refractive errors, ocular health, and functional vision, is part of a comprehensive visual assessment. For vision impairment to be properly diagnosed and managed, a comprehensive strategy is necessary.

A visual acuity evaluation measures a person's ability to see clearly and sharply at various distances. It is commonly carried out using charts such as the Snellen chart. This first stage aids in the identification of common refractive problems such as astigmatism, hyperopia, and myopia. The main source of vision impairment, refractive errors, can frequently be addressed with prescription glasses or contact lenses.

A thorough evaluation looks at the health of the eyes in addition to visual acuity. This entails examining the anterior and posterior segments of the eye with tools such as the slit-lamp biomicroscope. Examining the condition of the cornea, lens, and vitreous, special attention is paid to any anomalies or indications of eye disorders.

Imaging methods such as fundus photography and optical coherence tomography (OCT) are vital in evaluating the structural integrity of the retina and optic nerve. These instruments offer precise, high-resolution pictures of the retinal layers, which help with the identification of diseases like glaucoma, diabetic retinopathy, and macular degeneration.

Beyond a physical examination, a functional vision assessment measures an individual's ability to use their eyesight for everyday tasks. This entails evaluating color vision, depth perception, eye coordination, and visual field. Children should undergo functional vision testing to detect any visual impairments that can affect their development and ability to learn.

Comprehensive visual evaluations are not just for people who already have vision problems. For people of all ages, routine eye exams help with preventive care by identifying any problems before they manifest symptoms. Healthcare practitioners can customize interventions and treatment plans to address particular visual issues and promote overall eye health by utilizing a combination of diagnostic tools and approaches. To overcome vision impairment and improve the quality of life for people of all ages, a proactive and thorough approach to visual screening is important.

CHAPTER FIVE

OPTIONS FOR TREATMENT
Medical Procedures:

The goal of medical treatments for visual impairment is to treat underlying issues and disorders that impair vision. Medications are frequently used in these interventions to treat illnesses or ailments that worsen vision. For instance, medicine may be necessary for disorders like macular degeneration, diabetic retinopathy, or glaucoma to regulate blood sugar levels, reduce intraocular pressure, or delay the disease's progression.

Medicinal therapies for refractive defects, such as astigmatism, hyperopia, or myopia, typically involve prescription glasses or contact lenses. The inability of the eye to naturally refocus light onto the retina is compensated for by these corrective lenses. To evaluate changes in visual acuity and make necessary prescription adjustments, routine eye exams are vital.

Furthermore, pharmaceutical research advances have facilitated the creation of drugs that specifically target eye disorders. Anti-VEGF medications, for example, prevent the development of aberrant blood vessels in the retina and are used to treat wet age-related macular degeneration. For those with a variety of visual impairments, these medical therapies, when carried out under the supervision of a professional, can greatly improve or stabilize eyesight.

Surgical Techniques:

When medicinal interventions alone may not be adequate to correct vision impairment, surgical techniques become increasingly important. One of the most popular surgical treatments used to restore vision is cataract surgery. An artificial intraocular lens is used to replace the clouded natural lens during this treatment, improving vision clarity.

For those with injuries or illnesses of the cornea, another surgical option is corneal transplantation. To restore eyesight, a healthy donor cornea is used to replace the damaged or diseased cornea. Refractive errors are frequently corrected by laser eye surgery, such as LASIK or PRK, which reshapes the cornea and lessens the need for glasses or contact lenses.

Conditions such as vitreous hemorrhage or retinal detachment may necessitate retinal surgery. To stop more vision loss, surgeons can repair the detached retina or treat vitreous humor bleeding. Because these surgical treatments call for specific knowledge and tools, it is crucial to seek professional advice to get the best possible results.

Programs for Vision Rehabilitation:

The goal of vision rehabilitation programs is to optimize residual eyesight and improve the general quality of life for visually impaired people. These programs, which are frequently customized to meet the needs of the individual, include a variety of services like education on activities of daily living, mobility and orientation, and training on adapted technology.

With the use of methods like working with guide dogs or utilizing a white cane, orientation, and mobility training teaches people how to properly traverse their surroundings. Learning how to use tools and software like screen readers, software for magnifying images, and braille displays—which are intended to help people with visual impairments—is known as adaptive technology training.

Additionally, counseling and support groups may be a part of vision rehabilitation programs to treat the psychological and emotional components of visual impairment. Adaptive methods and coping strategies are essential elements that enable people to preserve their freedom and confidently participate in everyday activities.

Therapeutic Strategies:

A range of non-invasive methods are used in treatments for visual impairment to enhance visual function and lessen the effects of vision loss on day-to-day functioning. For example, vision therapy includes a range of exercises and activities intended to improve visual skills like depth perception, eye coordination, and attention. Conditions like strabismus (crossed eyes) and amblyopia (lazy eye) benefit most from it.

Another therapy strategy that concentrates on making the most of residual eyesight is low-vision rehabilitation. To maximize visual functioning, specialist optical instruments like telescopes, magnifiers, or electronic aids are prescribed. Occupational therapists are vital in the rehabilitation of people with impaired vision because they help patients modify their living and working situations to better meet their visual demands.

Apart from this, complementary and alternative methods such as nutritional therapy and acupuncture are becoming more popular for treating certain eye disorders. Some patients report subjective improvements in their visual function after adding these complementary therapies to their treatment plans, although research on the effectiveness of these approaches is still underway.

The choice of therapy modalities is frequently based on an individual's specific visual impairment, underlying causes, and special requirements. Working together with a group of medical specialists, such as occupational therapists, rehabilitation specialists, and optometrists, guarantees a thorough and customized treatment plan to overcome visual impairment.

CHAPTER SIX

ASSISTIVE TECHNOLOGY FOR EYE PROBLEMS
Assistive Technology Overview:

Helping people who are blind or visually impaired is a major responsibility of assistive technologies, which provide creative ways to increase their freedom and usability in many areas of life. With the help of tools and resources, these technologies aim to close the gap that exists between the visually impaired and the visual world, facilitating daily activities, education, and employment. The main objective is to establish a welcoming atmosphere where people with vision impairments can prosper and actively engage in society.

A vast array of hardware and software are included in assistive technologies, which meet a variety of needs and preferences. Screen readers, braille displays, software for magnification, and smart gadgets are a few examples of the categories into which these technologies might be divided.

Every category focuses on certain issues that people with visual impairments encounter and provides specialized solutions to enhance their overall quality of life.

Displays in Braille and Screen Readers:

In the field of assistive technologies for visual impairment, screen readers and braille displays are essential components. Software programs known as screen readers translate text on a computer or mobile device screen into synthetic voice. Users may now connect with apps, browse digital content, and get information thanks to this. On the other side, braille displays offer a tactile interface that enables people to read and understand information through touch by converting digital text into braille characters.

These tools make it possible for visually impaired people to pursue professional and educational goals, interact with digital content, and engage in a society that is heavily reliant on technology. Screen readers and braille displays work together seamlessly to improve accessibility, which makes internet content, documents, and applications more usable for those with vision problems.

Magnification Tools and Software:

To meet the demands of people with limited vision, assistive technologies can benefit from the addition of hardware and software that magnifies objects. With the help of these tools, users with visual impairments can view and navigate content more easily by enlarging text, images, and interface components on screens. Magnification software makes it possible for people with limited vision to comfortably connect with digital devices and take part in a variety of activities, such as reading, writing, and internet browsing, by improving visual aspects.

These technologies enhance professional and educational settings in addition to helping with everyday duties. Professionals can effectively use digital tools and traverse complex papers, while students can access textbooks, read lecture notes, and do research. The accessibility of the digital world for those with vision impairments is greatly enhanced by the adaptability of devices and software for magnification.

Smart Apps and Devices:

The way people with visual impairments engage with the world around them has been completely transformed by the integration of smart gadgets and apps. With the help of specialist apps and accessibility features, users of smartphones, tablets, and wearable technology may do a wide range of tasks on their own. Smart devices provide an extensive set of capabilities to improve communication, navigation, and information access. These tools range from using voice commands and gesture controls to accessing location-based information and using image recognition to identify things.

These devices encourage social inclusion in addition to independence. While communication apps enable smooth communication with others, navigation applications offer real-time direction, enabling users to confidently navigate unfamiliar settings. The ongoing creation of cutting-edge applications catered to the unique requirements of people with visual impairments guarantees their ability to remain involved, informed, and connected in the digital era. The ability of technology to break down barriers for people with visual impairments and open doors for a more inclusive and accessible future is best demonstrated by smart gadgets and apps.

CHAPTER SEVEN

SUPPORT FOR EDUCATION AND INCLUSIVE APPROACHES
Education that is Inclusive for Visual Impairment:

One of the most important components of developing a learning environment that meets the various needs of every student is inclusive education for visual impairment. By integrating visually impaired children into regular classes, inclusionists provide a setting in which they can learn alongside their peers without encountering prejudice or exclusion.

This method helps kids become more socially adept, develop empathy, and get ready for encounters in the real world. Beyond simple physical integration, inclusive education entails modifying curricula, evaluations, and teaching strategies to enable visually impaired students to engage fully in class and achieve academic success.

The foundation of effective inclusive education is a dedication to accessibility and the dismantling of obstacles, both structural and mental. Schools must make investments in tactile pathways and ramps, among other accessible infrastructure, to help visually impaired pupils move around more easily. To apply inclusive teaching practices and have a comprehensive grasp of the varied needs of children with visual impairments, educators should also complete training.

This could entail making adjustments to the instructional materials, utilizing assistive technology, and offering more help as needed. To ensure that educational experiences are customized to meet the specific requirements of each visually impaired student, collaboration between educators, parents, and experts is essential.

Additionally, encouraging an inclusive school culture makes children without visual impairments more happy. Students can cultivate empathy, compassion, and a willingness to work together with their peers who are visually impaired through awareness programs and sensitization. In addition to being an educational perspective, inclusive education for visual impairments includes a social commitment to accepting diversity and giving all pupils, regardless of ability, equal chances.

Classroom Setup:

Making necessary modifications in the classroom is essential to ensure that visually impaired students can engage completely in the educational process. To meet the specific needs of visually impaired students, these accommodations include a variety of tweaks and changes that support equitable access to educational programs. Having assistive technologies available in the classroom, like braille displays, screen readers, and software for magnification, is crucial for making reading and writing assignments easier. For visually challenged children, classrooms should also have good lighting and acoustics to improve the learning environment.

For visually impaired pupils, it is essential to make physical modifications to the classroom layout, such as thoughtful seating arrangements and well-defined walkways, to ensure their ease of mobility. Teachers ought to receive training on assisting visually impaired students in the classroom and directing them about as needed. Furthermore, by using various sensory channels to convey information, the utilization of tactile and aural cues might improve the learning process.

Customized Education Plans (IEPs) play a crucial role in ensuring that classroom adjustments are made to meet the unique requirements of every visually impaired student. These plans might include longer assessment times, different homework, and more help from resource teachers.

Educators, parents, and experts must have regular communication to assess the success of accommodations and make any required modifications. School districts may establish an inclusive learning environment where visually impaired children can succeed academically and socially by putting deliberate and comprehensive classroom adjustments into place.

Materials for Adaptive Learning:

For those who are visually impaired, adaptive learning resources are essential to a successful educational experience. To guarantee that visually impaired students have access to the same educational content as their sighted counterparts, these products are specifically made to meet the varied needs of these students.

The inclusion of tactile components in adaptive learning materials—such as tactile diagrams, 3D models, and braille books—is essential. Students who are blind or visually handicapped can interact with and understand difficult ideas in science, math, and geography thanks to these tactile resources.

Adaptive learning materials have been transformed by digital technology, which offers interactive and customized content.

Students with visual impairments can access and explore digital resources independently thanks to e-books that come with built-in accessibility features, audio descriptions, and screen reader compatibility. Additionally, adaptable programs and software can be customized to match the unique learning preferences of each user, resulting in a customized and inclusive learning environment.

Creating and executing adaptive learning resources requires cooperation between educators and experts. When it comes to choosing, producing, and applying these resources in the classroom, teachers require training. Furthermore, the field of adaptive technology continues to innovate and conduct research, which helps to improve learning resources for people with visual impairments.

Educational institutions may remove obstacles to learning, empower visually impaired students, and foster diversity in the classroom by investing in the creation and use of adapted learning resources.

<u>**Specific Instructional Strategies:**</u>

To guarantee that visually impaired students receive an excellent education that is customized to meet their specific learning needs, specialized teaching strategies are essential. To effectively handle the various problems presented by visual impairment, educators need to possess a repertory of tactics that extend beyond conventional teaching methods. Using multisensory techniques, which use several senses to deliver information, is one crucial technique. To reinforce concepts and improve understanding, instructors can, for instance, employ tactile items, auditory cues, and vocal descriptions.

A further essential element of customized instruction for visual impairment is differentiated instruction. Teachers must modify their teaching strategies to meet the needs of each visually impaired student because this demographic has a wide range of talents and learning preferences. To ensure maximum comprehension, this may entail giving more explanations, offering different forms for assignments, or modifying the pace of learning.

Effective specialized education requires collaboration with professionals, such as teachers in orientation and mobility, braille instructors, and assistive technology specialists. These experts can advise on how to use best practices as well as insights into the unique requirements of visually impaired students. Workshops, training sessions, and conferences are important forms of professional development for educators that help them become more proficient in particular teaching methods.

Furthermore, the success of specialized teaching methods depends critically on creating a welcoming and happy classroom environment. Teachers should foster teamwork, peer support, and an atmosphere where students feel comfortable asking for help. Through the use of customized teaching methods, educators may help visually impaired students reach their full potential, developing a passion for studying and giving them the confidence to overcome obstacles in their academic path.

CHAPTER EIGHT

ASPECTS OF VISUAL IMPAIRMENT THAT ARE PSYCHOSOCIAL
Personal Emotional Effects:

Visually impaired people may experience significant emotional consequences that touch different facets of their lives. Grief is frequently one of the main feelings felt, as people lament the loss of their vision and the way of life they used to lead. Living with a visual impairment can be difficult to adjust to, and it can cause frustration, rage, and even sadness. The person is not the only one affected emotionally; daily encounters and intimate connections are also impacted.

Many problems with self-esteem can also arise from having a visual impairment. People may experience a loss of independence and competence, as well as a weakened sense of self-worth. People who experience visual impairment may internalize unfavorable perceptions and suffer from a sense of belonging, which can be made worse by the cultural stigma attached to the condition. To promote resilience and enable people to accept their abilities beyond their physical constraints, it becomes imperative to address these mental difficulties.

Furthermore, a typical emotional reaction to visual impairment is anxiety. Elevated anxiety levels can be caused by a fear of the unknown, anxieties about safety, and difficulties navigating the environment. People may also struggle with anticipatory anxiety associated with social situations and the possibility of misinterpretation or condemnation. It's critical to identify and deal with these emotional reactions to support general well-being and assist in adjusting to visual impairment.

It is crucial to take into account holistic strategies, such as support groups and psychiatric counseling while managing the emotional impact. These therapies can offer a secure setting where people can express their feelings, create coping mechanisms, and strengthen their resilience. In addition, cultivating self-compassion and an optimistic outlook can greatly lessen the emotional toll that visual impairment has on a person, empowering them to overcome their emotional obstacles with more resilience and flexibility.

Adaptive Techniques:

People with visual impairments frequently use a range of coping mechanisms to get through the difficulties posed by their changed surroundings. There are several categories into which coping strategies can be divided, such as emotion- and problem-focused coping. The practical components of visual impairment are addressed through problem-focused coping, which includes obtaining assistive equipment and learning adaptive skills to improve day-to-day functioning.

Acquiring new abilities, including mobility training and orientation, can empower those who are visually impaired. These abilities not only promote more independence but also build self-assurance when interacting with the outside world. In contrast, emotion-focused coping focuses on controlling one's emotional reactions to vision loss. This can entail asking friends, relatives, or mental health specialists for emotional assistance.

Participating in leisure pursuits tailored for those with visual impairments can also be an effective coping mechanism. Engaging in sports, the arts, or other recreational pursuits modified to meet visual impairments promotes a feeling of belonging and normalcy. In addition to being enjoyable, these activities support the growth of a positive identity that transcends the limitations of visual impairment.

Developing a resilient attitude is also an important coping mechanism. Positivity can be enhanced by motivating people to celebrate their accomplishments, set reasonable goals, and concentrate on their strengths. Building a toolkit of coping mechanisms based on personal preferences and requirements is essential because it helps people to actively handle the difficulties brought on by visual impairment and continue to lead meaningful lives.

Putting Together a Support Network:

Creating a strong support network is crucial for people who are managing visual impairment. It is not a trip that should be traveled alone, and having a network of supporters can have a big impact on a person's overall quality of life and emotional health. The support system can take many forms, such as friends, family, medical experts, and neighborhood organizations that focus on vision impairment.

Family is an important source of both practical and emotional support. Families need to communicate openly to voice worries, anxieties, and requirements about vision impairment. Family members can also help an individual adapt by creating a welcoming and cheerful atmosphere.

Having friends and social connections are both crucial for creating a network of support. Keeping up social ties promotes a sense of belonging and helps fight feelings of isolation. Creating an inclusive social circle, promoting empathy, and educating friends about visual impairment are all crucial elements of creating a network of supportive peers.

An essential component of the support system consists of medical professionals such as ophthalmologists, rehabilitation specialists, and mental health practitioners. Individuals with visual impairment benefit from regular check-ups, psychological support, and access to rehabilitation treatments. Working together, the patient and medical staff may guarantee a thorough and customized approach to controlling vision impairment.

In addition to increased resources, community organizations, and support groups that are expressly focused on visual impairment provide a sense of community. These organizations give people a place to talk about their experiences, trade coping mechanisms, and get useful information. By becoming a part of these groups, people can develop a feeling of community and strength from one another when overcoming the obstacles associated with vision impairment.

In summary, creating a support system is a dynamic, continuous process that necessitates the active participation of numerous stakeholders. In addition to aiding with the psychological effects of vision loss, a strong support network is essential for assisting people in learning healthy coping mechanisms and leading happy lives despite obstacles they may face.

CHAPTER NINE

LIVING INDEPENDENTLY WITH VISUAL IMPAIRMENT
Adaptive Living Skills:

Developing and perfecting adapted living skills is necessary for living independently with a visual impairment. These abilities are essential for completing everyday tasks and routines. These abilities cover a wide range, such as efficient communication, organization, and personal care, among others. People who are visually impaired need to learn how to recognize and navigate their environment through assistive technology or tactile approaches. Gaining adapted living skills is a multifaceted process that calls for instruction in several areas.

Personal care is an important component, where people learn how to take care of their hygiene, clothing, and grooming. This entails labeling personal belongings, utilizing tactile clues, and making use of adapting devices like talking watches or braille labels. Additionally, effective work management requires strong organizational abilities. Important strategies include using tactile markers or utilizing accessible technologies for reminders and scheduling.

A further essential adaptive ability is communication. To improve their communication skills, people with visual impairment frequently pick up alternate techniques like braille, auditory clues, or computerized voice assistants. Along with encouraging independence, these abilities also help people become more self-assured and self-sufficient.

Mobility training and orientation: For people with visual impairments who want to live independently, mobility training and orientation are essential. To confidently navigate both interior and outdoor settings, this training focuses on developing spatial awareness, comprehending environmental cues, and mastering mobility strategies. Orientation and mobility teachers assist people in creating a mental map of their environment that integrates both tactile and aural cues.

Using landmarks, adjusting to environmental changes, and becoming proficient at moving around a living area are all part of indoor navigation. On the other hand, outdoor mobility entails learning how to navigate streets, take public transportation, and recognize directional cues from sounds and surrounding elements.

Beyond merely teaching movement, orientation, and mobility training also includes teaching problem-solving techniques to deal with unforeseen obstacles. Gaining these abilities helps people with visual impairment feel more independent and free, which enhances their capacity to interact with the outside world in ways that suit them.

Modifications to the Home:

It is essential to provide a home setting that supports independent living for visually impaired individuals. Making necessary changes to a home is essential to creating a secure and usable living environment. This entails modifying the actual surroundings to meet the special requirements and difficulties that come with visual impairment.

Simple improvements like appropriate lighting and color contrast can be made, as can larger ones like adding tactile flooring, handrails, or ramps. The purpose of these modifications is to improve the person's capacity to move around their house with assurance and autonomy.

Technology also has a big impact on home modifications. Smart home appliances, for example, boost accessibility by using voice commands and automation.

Adapting the house to each person's unique needs promotes a feeling of empowerment and security. It gives visually impaired people the ability to carry out everyday tasks with less help, encouraging a higher level of independence.

Employment & Career Guidance: Having a rewarding career is not just financially necessary for people with visual impairments, but it's also a route to personal development and empowerment. To remove barriers in the workplace, persons with visual impairments must receive employment and career coaching tailored to their specific needs.

This advice entails determining appropriate career pathways, offering adaptive technology training, and cultivating skills that meet the needs of the selected field. Vocational rehabilitation services, which provide training in job interview techniques, resume construction, and workplace adaption, are essential in helping people with visual impairments.

One important factor to consider is accessibility in the workplace. To guarantee a welcoming workplace, employers can provide accommodations like screen readers, software for magnification, or accessible papers. Furthermore, visually impaired people can benefit from networking opportunities and mentoring programs that offer a supportive group as well as insightful guidance on navigating the professional world.

With focused job placement and career coaching, people with visual impairments can overcome obstacles, seek fulfilling jobs, and actively participate in the workforce. This breaks down social stereotypes about the ability of people with visual impairments in the workplace and encourages financial independence.

CHAPTER TEN

TRIUMPHANT TALES AND MOTIVATIONAL TRAVELS
Profiles of People Getting Over Vision Impairment

Many people have become inspirational figures in the field of overcoming vision impairment, demonstrating that tenacity and willpower can overcome obstacles of a physical nature. Emily Turner is one such extraordinary person who, despite receiving a diagnosis of a degenerative eye disease at an early age, refused to allow her vision handicap to limit her potential.

Having a strong interest in technology since childhood, Emily explored the world of software and assistive gadgets that could give her more power. She adopted adaptive technologies under the advice of subject-matter specialists, which enabled her to complete a computer science degree and establish herself as a prominent voice for inclusive technology.

The inspiring tale of visually handicapped athlete Michael Rodriguez, who defied social expectations to succeed in athletics, is another. Michael's genetic problem caused him to lose his vision, but it didn't stop him from following his passion for sports. He developed his para-athletic abilities with the help of knowledgeable trainers and adaptive sports programs, eventually participating in the Paralympic Games. Michael's story dispels myths about athletics and handicaps while also emphasizing the value of professional assistance while adjusting to new physical pursuits.

The variety of experiences within the visually challenged people is exemplified by these anecdotes. While some overcome obstacles to education and go on to have successful jobs through mentorship and adaptive technologies, others overcome physical constraints to become elite athletes. All of these people have one thing in common: they were given crucial advice by professionals who are aware of the complexities of vision impairment and who enable them to function in a world where sight is everything.

Accomplishments in Multiple Domains

Beyond individual victories, the success stories of people who have overcome vision disability are widespread in a variety of professional domains. Sarah Johnson is a very successful lawyer who chose to practice law even though she had a progressive vision loss problem. Sarah became a trailblazer in fighting for inclusive legal proccdures, in addition to navigating the difficulties of law school, with the guidance of seasoned legal practitioners who recognized the value of accessibility. Her experience highlights how crucial professional advice is in breaking down barriers in the workplace.

Within the field of arts and entertainment, the narrative of vision-handicapped musician Alex Chen is very captivating. Under the guidance of professionals in the field of music accessibility, Alex made use of cutting-edge methods and tools to keep following his love of writing music. His compositions, which fuse aspects of the classical and modern styles, have not only won praise from critics but also disproved notions regarding the constraints of vision impairment in the creative domain.

These accomplishments highlight how professional supervision can enable people with visual impairments to achieve success in a variety of industries. Collaboration between individuals and experienced mentors can enable the creation and implementation of adaptive methods in various professional fields, such as law or music. This can lead to a more inclusive and accessible environment for all.

CHAPTER ELEVEN

FUTURE DIRECTIONS AND RESEARCH DEVELOPMENTS IN MEDICINE:

Recent years have seen notable advancements in the field of medical research targeted at providing professional help to overcome visual impairment. There are now more options for comprehending and treating a range of visual impairments thanks to the investigation of cutting-edge technologies and creative methods. Researchers studying the genetics of inherited vision problems are making significant progress in the field of gene therapy. Medical researchers want to create tailored therapies that can potentially reverse or halt the course of disorders like macular degeneration and retinitis pigmentosa by identifying and correcting specific genetic abnormalities causing these deficits.

Moreover, a new treatment option for visual impairment has been made possible by the development of stem cell research. Researchers are looking into how stem cells might regenerate damaged or degraded retinal cells. This method may be useful in situations where vision impairment is caused by irreversible cell loss.

The safety and effectiveness of stem cell therapies are being evaluated through clinical studies and research, which is a revolutionary step in the fight to recover vision.

Neurotechnologies are being used in addition to genetic and cellular therapies to circumvent impaired visual circuits and restore vision. Optic nerve stimulation and brain-computer interfaces are being researched as viable ways to close the gap between vision impairment and visual perception.

These novel methods give hope to patients with disorders affecting the pathways involved in visual processing, either by decoding visual information straight from the brain or by electrically stimulating the optic nerve to convey signals to the brain.

Emerging Assistive Technologies:

The field of assistive technologies, which are meant to help visually impaired people, is changing quickly. Current advancements concentrate on giving users a more thorough and customized experience in addition to improving accessibility. These advancements would not be possible without artificial intelligence (AI) and machine learning, which allow gadgets to adjust to the unique requirements of each user. Wearers of smart glasses with computer vision capabilities can get real-time information by having the glasses recognize and describe objects, text, and even people.

Developments in haptic technology, which transmits information through touch feedback, have also been essential in producing more immersive assistive technology. Users of wearable technology that incorporates tactile feedback methods can "feel" images and visuals, which enhances their perception of their environment. Furthermore, navigation systems with sound-based cues and 3D spatial mapping allow visually impaired people to navigate unknown areas with confidence.

Furthermore, new opportunities for improving the recreational and educational experiences of people with visual impairments have been made possible by the integration of augmented reality (AR) and virtual reality (VR) technologies. AR and VR-created immersive environments can imitate a variety of circumstances, offering useful training possibilities and encouraging hands-on learning. In addition to being helpful tools, these technologies also improve the general well-being and social inclusion of those who are visually impaired.

Positive Approaches to Education:

Promising educational techniques are part of the efforts to fight visual impairment with professional assistance, which goes beyond medical and technical solutions. Models of inclusive education that emphasize integrating students with visual impairments into regular classrooms are becoming more and more popular. These approaches place a high priority on establishing a welcoming classroom with teachers who are prepared to meet the requirements of students with varying learning styles.

Accessible learning material innovations are essential to providing visually impaired students with an equal playing field. Curriculum developers are using tactile graphics, audiobooks, and braille displays to make sure that all students can access the material. Furthermore, developments in assistive technologies have permeated the educational field, providing students with visual impairments with resources such as voice recognition software, screen readers, and adaptive learning environments.

Moreover, there is an increasing focus on creating customized educational curricula that are tailored to the particular learning needs of people who are blind or visually impaired. These programs emphasize social integration, independence, and the development of critical life skills in addition to academic courses.

Effective educational methods that enable people with visual impairments to reach their full potential are designed and implemented via the collaborative efforts of educators, rehabilitation specialists, and assistive technology experts.

In conclusion, overcoming vision impairment is not only a possibility but also a goal that will be attained in the future thanks to the combined efforts of medical research, developing assistive technologies, and promising educational approaches. These many strategies highlight the value of an all-encompassing, multidisciplinary strategy in addressing the intricate problems related to vision impairment. To open up new avenues and enhance the lives of those who are visually impaired, researchers, technologists, educators, and healthcare professionals must continue to collaborate.